# Reiki For Beginners:

How to Relax, Reduce Stress, and Increase your Energy

through the Power of Reiki

## Table of Contents

# Introduction

Man has been healing others since the beginning of time, as there has been a healing agent available in the invisible realm the entire time. See, at the core of the universe everything is energy. This energy is extremely powerful and useful for humankind in a variety of ways.

Before we get into the depths of Reiki, let's look at Reiki through a practical, tangible example that you can experience right away.

The idea of Reiki is that all through the universe there is a vibration or a frequency that permeates all things, including the stars, planets, humans, animals, plants, rocks, and even the air and water. Liken it to the Force from Star Wars. Imagine that anything that makes you feel upset or stressed out as static or a disturbance in the energy flowing through your mind and body. This harmonic frequency of the universe is vibrating very fast and can cause any slower, unhealthy vibrations you are having to attune to it such an amazing power so that you can feel happy and healthy.

If you know how to attune yourself to that energy and allow it to flow through your mind and body, it can make the static that makes you unhappy or feeling stressed harmonize. Ultimately, if that contended with, your body can heal the way it is supposed to heal.

This is the essence of Reiki.

It isn't magical or mystical any more than your cell phone is magical or mystical. It might be *mysterious* to you right now but this is because you do not fully understand it yet. As your understanding grows, so will your ability to use it.

Gratitude is the way

What really gets Reiki energy flowing nicely is gratitude, as gratitude is the ultimate teacher of Reiki vibrations. Think of tuning in a radio station and the difference a minute change will cause in the radio frequency and how easily you can hear the music or the static between frequencies. If you can really tune into Reiki, you will find it much easier to manipulate this energy.

Most Reiki masters will tell you that Reiki is a benevolent 'love' energy. This is a wonderful way to describe it. It encompasses gratitude, love, happiness and joy – all positive emotions. A simple way to put yourself into this mindset is to think about a person you feel gratitude or thankfulness toward. He or she will be someone that has done or said something to help you or somehow conferred a benefit upon you. This will help you to begin thinking positively, which is necessary to begin feeling the Reiki energy flowing through you.

Let's perform a short exercise to let you feel what this energy is like when you concentrate and let it manifest. You will learn more about these steps later on in this book.

- Take a deep breath in.

- Breathe out.

- Take another deep breath in.

- And breathe out again.

- Call to mind someone you are grateful toward.

  - This is someone who has been very kind, loving and generous toward you.

- Lift your hands in front of you, palm up and about chest or belly high.

- Invite the essence or spirit of that person into your hands.

  - Reflect upon that person and all that they mean to you.

  - Consider how your hands feel as you are holding this person's essence in your hands.

  - You may feel your hands beginning to tingle or getting warmer.

Did you feel your hands beginning to tingle? This is how you can really connect with the healing energy associated with Reiki. You may notice that when you are in that moment of gratitude that you cannot hold an angry feeling. Gratitude and anger cannot be held in the same place at the same time.

Envision the flow

Visualization is powerful. Go ahead and envision that there is white light in the universe that is flowing through you. Envision this power to enter the crown of your head, wash down the back of your neck, through your shoulders, upper arms, forearms and coming out and extending out through your hands.

By now you should be feeling a tingle and/or a warmth in your hands. Imagine your hands being able to harmonize with the things that you touch.

- Move your hands to the sides of your face.

- Feel the warmth entering your cheeks from your hands.

- Know that this calm and restorative energy can flow through you and wash through your skin and out through your feet.

This is how you can connect to the energy that is Reiki. The following chapters will give you the information about Reiki and a more in-depth exploration into how you can experience the energy of Reiki to help you to relax, reduce your stress levels and increase your natural energy.

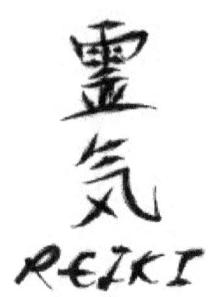

REIKI

## Just what is Reiki?

Reiki, pronounced *ray-key*, is a form of energy healing that manipulates the energy that flows through your body naturally. Your entire body at its core is made up of vibrating energy. You may be entirely skeptical that such a thing as this 'spiritual life force energy' could even exist. Whether it exists or not, *something* exists within your body to cause an electrical force that allows synapses to fire within your brain, pain signals to pass from your brain to your muscles, then back again. In addition to this, some kind of electrical communication is happening between muscles without even going to the brain!

Doctors know there is energy inside the body

Doctors use *electro*encephalographs (EEGs) to check the energy used by your brain, *electro*cardiograms (ECGs) to be sure your heart is working right and *electro*myography (EMGs) to see if your muscles are communicating with your nerves correctly and how fast those messages are passing.

Why can't there be some kind of life force flowing through your body that can be manipulated by someone practicing this type of energy healing?

Now, you might be thinking that Reiki is some kind of religious cult since I've mentioned it being a 'spiritual life force', but it really isn't. You don't have to believe in *anything* other than what you really want to believe.

Reiki is used by many cultures

Reiki is practiced by people of all types of religion, as well as those with no religious beliefs. If there is anything 'religious' about Reiki, it is that you must *believe* it will work for you!

Some may not believe that just waving your hands over your body can alter the natural energy flow, but it is quite true and possible. Some practitioners can do this, but many modern Reiki therapists use actual massage to help to restore the natural flow of that energy within your body. You can learn how to do that too! I know that if I hurt somewhere, the pain will just keep roiling up that energy just like big rocks in the middle of a river creates a series of rapids.

Imagine you're in a raft on a nice placid river, just floating along. You hear a low rumbling just at the edge of your hearing and when you travel around the bend in the river, there ahead of you is a set of rapids. Some rapids just make your raft bounce around a little but others can make your raft bounce, dip and spin around because the flow of the water is so disrupted by the rocks beneath the surface. Muscle pain causes these same disturbances in that energy flowing through your body, so the Reiki therapist will sometimes use regular massage techniques to ease the pain. They can then encourage that life force to flow more smoothly to take healing to the part of the body that needs it.

Reiki is not difficult to understand and it is quite easy to perform. Reiki is the use of the life force energy that occurs naturally in your body to heal your body through the belief that it will work *and* that the manipulation of your life force energy will facilitate that healing.

Read on to find out just how Reiki works.

# How does Reiki work?

Now that you know what Reiki is, the next step is to find out just how it works. Essentially, Reiki involves manipulation of your life force energy but isn't the actual life force energy. Confused yet? That's perfectly fine. Let's look at it in a different way and see if I can't clear up your confusion.

Your heart works through the contraction and relaxation of muscles stimulated by an electrical charge that keeps your heartbeat smooth and regular. If something is out of kilter in your heart and the electrical charges don't work right, a doctor may prescribe medications or surgically install tiny machines that assist in keeping those synapses between the muscles of your heart firing properly. Those are the pacemakers or defibrillators you hear about people having implanted. But if your heart stops, a 'crash cart' or defibrillator paddles are used to start it again by sending a jolt of electricity from an outside source through it.

The Energy Meridians

Your body at the core has energy meridians that flow through it. The following image is a diagram of how energies run through your body and the directions these energy currents run. The different meridian channels affect different portions of your body. The meridian line that runs from the crown of your head touches all of the other channels producing a conjunction where two lines intersect.  Which is why simply following the main line from crown to core (the base of your spine) will allow you to smooth out those auxiliary lines at the same time.

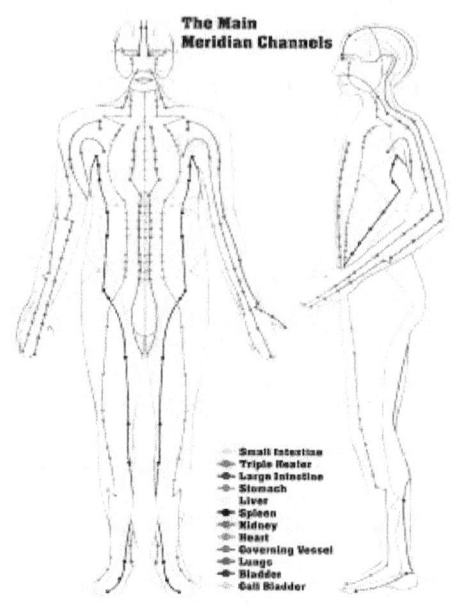

The Main Meridian Channels

Small Intestine
Triple Healer
Large Intestine
Stomach
Liver
Spleen
Kidney
Heart
Governing Vessel
Lungs
Bladder
Gall Bladder

Reiki works on that same principle since it is usually performed by a practitioner on a patient. The role of patient is pretty self-explanatory, while the practitioner is the outside source that is smoothing out those rapids in your life force energy we talked about earlier. Those ripples, knots, and blocks in the energy flow is what's causing you to feel unwell.

Life Force sustains you

Therapists who practice Reiki say that you are alive because of the life force flowing through you. This life force moves along paths or channels in your body that are commonly called chakras, meridians, or nadis. This life force runs through all the organs and cells of your body providing nourishment and support for all the functions carried out within each system.

The life force in your body can affect your health in both positive and negative ways through the thoughts and feelings you have about yourself. More specifically, the feelings about yourself in your subconscious mind that you may not be aware of having. The negative thoughts or feelings you have about yourself will cause ripples, eddies and knots in the flow of that energy causing you to feel physically unwell.

What a Reiki practitioner does is to introduce *positive* energy into those disturbed areas to 'charge' them to a point where the negative energies break up and just fall away. The slow, harmful vibrations become faster, healthier vibrations that help you feel better. When that happens, the positive energies used by the therapist smooth out your natural energies and whatever problem you were having will ease and finally disappear.

Reiki practitioners believe and will tell you that *they* are not guiding the healing but that the energy within you is doing what it already knows you need. The practitioner is just the conduit the energy is using to get past the blockages, or rapids, to get to where it needs to go. Therefore, even if Reiki doesn't work as well as you think it should for whatever problem you were, or are, having – it's not going to make the problem worse! That's reassuring, isn't it?

Come on! Let's see how Reiki can help you to relax.

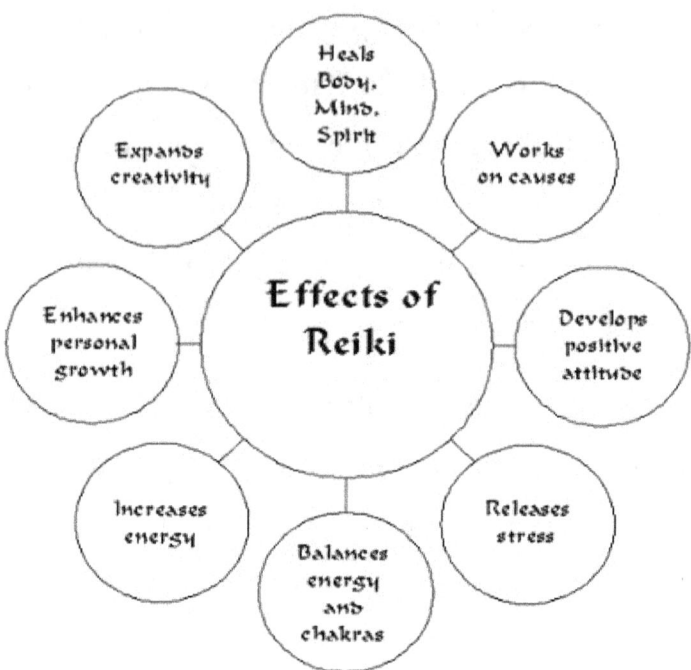

## Relaxing with Reiki.

Are you still skeptical that Reiki can actually help you relax? That's absolutely fine! You may already do relaxation techniques that let you think more clearly, work through knotty problems or just clear your mind and ease cramped muscles before you start or end your day. Reiki is just one more kind of relaxation technique you can employ to do all of those and much more.

You may be familiar with Yoga, deep breathing, biofeedback, meditation, Tai Chi or the devotions and prayers of your religious beliefs. Even walking, running, and gardening can be techniques that help you to relax and re-center yourself when you are feeling mentally tangled up.

As we discussed earlier, Reiki is simply manipulating the life force energy that flows through your body and this helps you relax. Just like the river flowing smoothly when there are no huge boulders near the surface, your life force energy will flow smoothly through your cells and organs. It will help you think more rationally and easily and you'll be able to make decisions more readily. Or perhaps you are anxious about a test you have to take or a speech you have been asked to make. Reiki will help with any anxiety you might feel in those situations.

## Reiki helps even when you don't expect it

Should everything be going quite well in your life, you might wonder how Reiki will be of help to you. When I heard about Reiki, I was in perfect health both physically and mentally so I wondered just how Reiki could help me. Actually, I found out that I was under stress and didn't even know it! All those little things you might not even think about put stress upon your body and mind causing little ripples in the energies that flows through you. It's just like one boulder near the surface of that smoothly flowing river disturbs the easy movement of the water.

## When it comes to doubts

When you have your first Reiki session, if you have some doubts about the treatment, it may not work as well as you think it should. This could be a result of your skepticism since mind over matter really is a bigger deal than most people think. It is important to believe that Reiki works in order to get the most out of the treatment. If you doubt, you are shorting yourself out of some great benefits, though you will certainly still getting some good energy flow. Even if you do not think you are getting results, you can be assured that it has had *some* result that will help you detect the effect of the process in your second Reiki treatment.

During your first session you may feel nothing physically but many have reported feeling warmth throughout their bodies no matter where the practitioner's hands are placed. Others have said they felt vibrations or just deep relaxation. The more accepting you are about the procedure, the more you will feel and be able to follow as your therapist performs the treatment. No matter what you feel, when the session is over, you will have a sense of well-being and refreshment with a more positive outlook on the world.

What to expect at the first session

Reiki practitioners want you to be comfortable so the process can be performed anywhere, though the quieter the surroundings, the better. Whomever you choose to receive a treatment from will be very attentive to your comfort and will not usually request any paperwork to be filled out like your personal physician may. The most you may have to do is sign a waiver giving them permission to perform the procedure. Most likely you will be asked if you have any health conditions that would interfere with your ability to lay flat on your back since Reiki works best when your body can completely relax.

The therapy room will probably look similar to a massage therapy room in many aspects, though the examination or treatment table won't necessarily have the hole for your face as a massage table does. If you aren't able to lay on your back then you may be asked to sit in a comfortable, supportive chair. You will not be asked to undress for your first session and subsequent treatments may or may not require partial or full disrobing, depending upon what you are receiving treatment for.

Music is often played to mask ambient sounds that might disturb you during your session. If you have a specific type of music that helps you relax or that you prefer when you meditate, you can usually request your Reiki therapist to play it during your procedure. Below is an example of how your therapy room may look. There is usually a single table rather than two unless you and a companion are receiving treatments together.

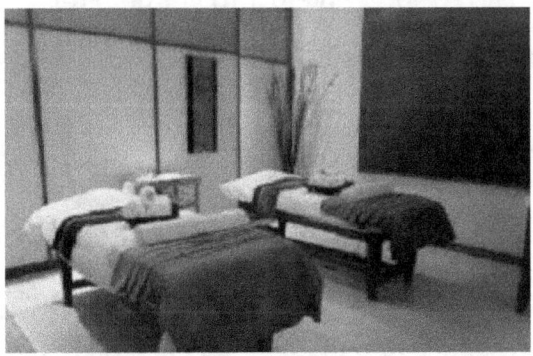

A normal Reiki session often consists of a light touch or hovering of the practitioner's hands on or over the head, face, front and back of your torso. The 6 chakra regions will be the primary focus, but the practitioner may focus on other areas as well if he feels led to do so. There is not usually any pressure brought to bear on those portions the therapist touches, similar to just resting your hand on those parts of your body. Your therapist will be conscientious about being sure that you do not experience physical or mental discomfort. The placement of the therapist's hands should never feel intrusive or inappropriate since this will cause adverse electrical impulses that will block the positive energy the Reiki attempts to impart.

As mentioned before, Reiki is simply a practitioner laying hands on portions of your body to help the energies contained within you to flow smoothly. However, some massage therapists are also trained and certified to practice Reiki and may incorporate both sets of training in any session after your first.

It may seem silly to go to someone just to get help relaxing, but without these types of techniques then you may not be fully relaxed. If you don't know how to do it on your own, then you need someone else to help you with it. When you find the person you want to give you Reiki, be sure to let them know everything that will make you comfortable. This is *your* special time and your therapist is there to make you feel wonderful. If you need a pillow beneath your knees or a blanket, if laying on your back or stomach is uncomfortable or if you don't care to be touched in specific places due to tender scar tissue from surgery or other physical injury – be sure to tell your therapist. It is their job to make you comfortable. If you are comfortable, the easier their job will be.

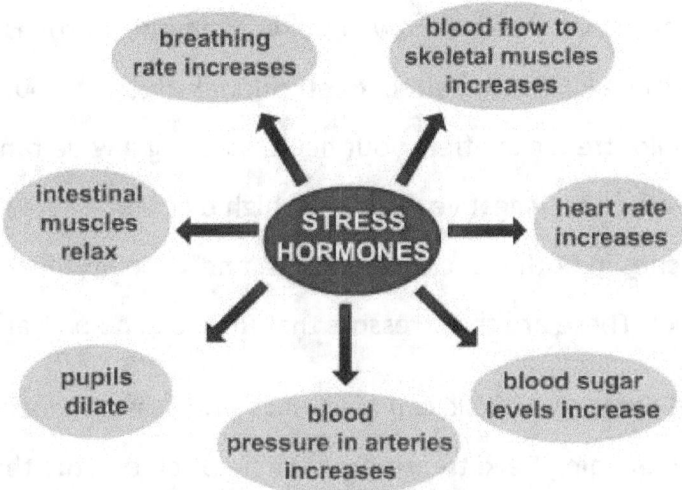

## Reiki reduces stress.

Stress is common in everyone's lives. In fact, according to many physicians, chronic stress is the cause of many ailments and illnesses. A little bit of stress may actually be beneficial, but too much is not. Good stress gives life zest! Getting married, having a child or getting a job promotion are all stressful, but they give a sense of fulfillment and enjoyment which are good. You might find yourself more social if you are under a bit of stress, like when you have to give a speech. You also might find that you trust people more and possibly be more creative. However, we are wanting to see how Reiki reduces stress and these types of stressors aren't the kind we want to reduce.

Chronic stress is stress that sticks with you for weeks, months, or even years. This is the stress you want to use Reiki to reduce so that it doesn't continue to affect your health or well-being. If anything proves the mind over matter of Reiki, it is the effect of emotional stress on your physical health. Chronic stress can affect your health causing a wide range of ailments: headaches, digestive problems, high blood pressure, heart problems, aches in both muscles and joints, and difficulty sleeping or staying awake. These are the stressors that Reiki can help to alleviate.

While a single session of Reiki can help you to relax and reduce stress immediately, ongoing Reiki treatments can help remove the thoughts or feelings that are behind those stressors. Think of multiple Reiki sessions as a form of therapy but instead of talking to your therapist, you are talking to yourself and the energy that flows within you. Reiki therapy is more in-depth than simply allowing a practitioner to smooth the flow of your energies. It requires a more active role from you than just as a passive recipient of the treatment.

When you choose to participate in Reiki therapy you will most likely be treated as a student who wishes to use Reiki to help others like yourself. Once you have learned to use Reiki, you can use it on yourself to continue reversing those thoughts and feelings you have about yourself to help reduce the stress in your life. It will also allow you to confront and deal with the new negative emotions you may encounter in the course of living.

Reiki is for everyone.

Anyone can learn Reiki. You don't have to have a high level of education, a psychic ability or even meditate as some religions require. What you do need to have is the belief that Reiki works, that it will work for you, and the acceptance that you can affect your own mind and body.

Along with the ability to help you relax and reduce stress, Reiki can increase your natural energy. Whether you have  decided to find a Reiki practitioner to perform the procedure for you or you have decided to learn it for yourself, you'll be amazed at how much more relaxed and energized you feel after your first session.

# Increase your Energy with Reiki

Oddly enough, improvement in your energy levels is actually a side effect of using Reiki. Since Reiki helps you relax and reduce stress, it will automatically increase your natural energy levels. Below is an image of an electromagnetic scan of a human body before and after using Reiki to smooth out the knots and wrinkles in the life force energy. Since it is an electromagnetic field natural to the body, it can be detected and measured with scientific instruments.

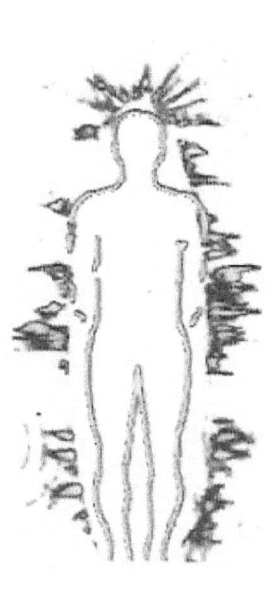 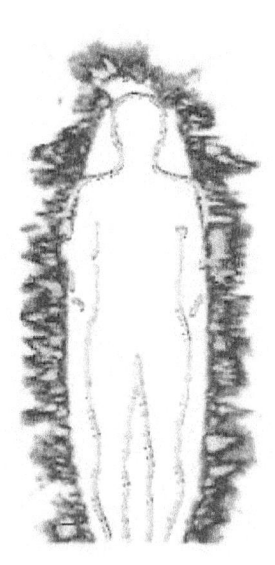

Stress can tear or puncture the energy field running around and through your body. It can also cause blockages. These injuries to your life force energy can cause both acute and chronic conditions to occur that disrupt your general health. The above image shows just how Reiki can help to heal those tears or punctures in that energy field and make it stronger.

The use of Reiki turns off or tones down your body's response to stressors because it takes a large amount of energy to maintain that fight or flight response. If your body is always in a state of agitation, you aren't going to have much energy to devote to anything else, are you?

That fight or flight response is brought about by stimulation of the adrenal glands that sit on top of your kidneys. Adrenaline is a hormone the adrenal glands secrete that gives you a jolt of energy that lets you either fight for your life or the energy to run away. They also secrete cortisol at the same time. Cortisol increases the glucose in the blood since glucose is broken down to provide energy to the muscles.

However, if you have constant secretion of adrenaline and cortisol this can result in higher blood pressure, increased heart rate and high blood glucose levels. If the glucose in your blood isn't made into energy then it is automatically made into fat which is usually deposited in your abdominal region. The increase in fat deposited in your body will increase your weight, which will decrease your energy level and increase the debilitating effects that low energy levels can cause.

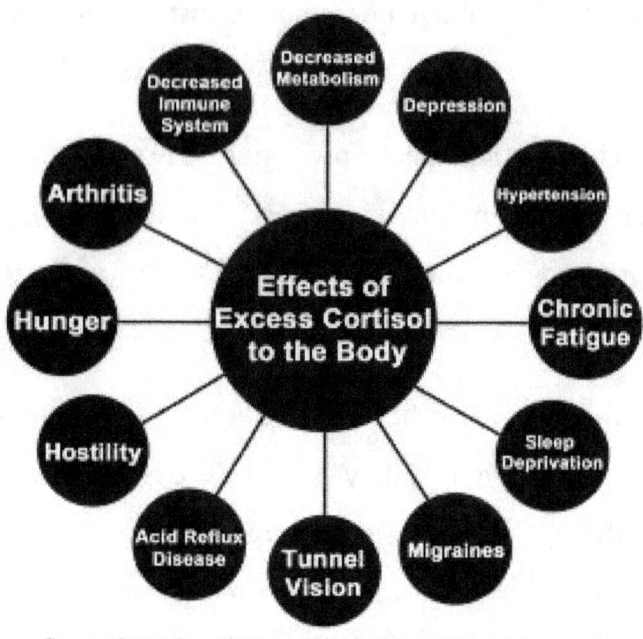

## Cortisol - The Stress Hormone

Low energy levels can also make it more difficult for you to sleep, or to stay awake. I know it sounds confusing but they are actually related. If you are stressed about something, you may not be able to sleep because your mind will go round and round not allowing you to relax enough to sleep. Since you aren't sleeping well, when you wake up you will most likely be tired all day and may find it difficult to remain awake.

The use of Reiki will increase your energy to allow you to fall asleep more easily, sleep deeper and longer, and to awake refreshed. Since you will be sleeping better, you aren't going to find yourself needing that pot of coffee in the morning just to be able to function or wanting to take a power nap just to be able to finish off your shift at work.

Since you will be sleeping better and having a higher level of that natural energy flowing through your body, you will find that you can think more clearly and make more rational decisions. That mental clarity can make you less mentally exhausted since you won't have to work as hard to piece thoughts together.

Now, I know that I have talked a lot about how Reiki can help you and about Reiki therapists and sessions. But what if the budget is tighter than a cork stuck in a bottle? Well, relax! Yes, that pun was intended. You don't have to shell out a lot of money to get the benefits of Reiki. Like I said before, *anyone* can learn Reiki. Even you.

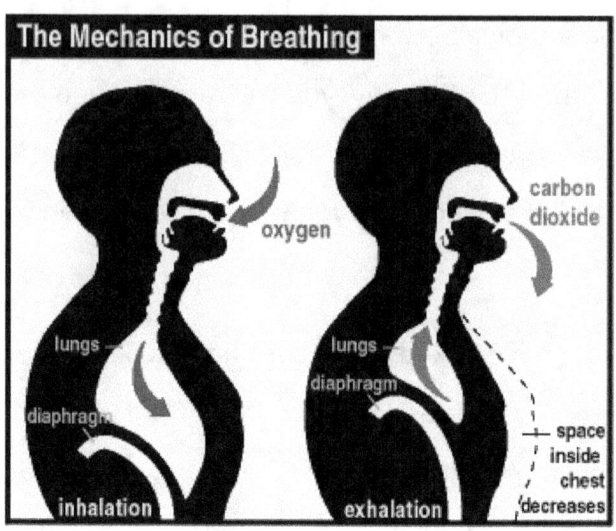

**The Mechanics of Breathing**

oxygen

carbon dioxide

lungs

diaphragm

lungs

diaphragm

space inside chest decreases

inhalation

exhalation

## Breathing: It really is Important!

Yes, I know … if you aren't breathing, then you aren't alive. But have you ever really just *breathed*? I mean, *really* paid attention to it? If you haven't, take a few minutes and do it now.

Just sit where you are. If you're in a straight backed chair, lift your chin so it's parallel to the floor and pull your shoulders back just a little to align your spine and open your rib cage and abdomen. Let your hands rest on your thighs as you maintain that position and just relax your muscles as much as you can. Now close your eyes.

Inhale through your nose for a count of four: one-one thousand, two-one thousand, three-one thousand, four-one thousand. Some people can inhale longer than four seconds. If you are one of those lucky people, inhale as you count the seconds until you can't inhale any more.

Feel how your shoulders lift as you pull that breath in. Feel your rib cage expanding, the cartilage between those slender bones stretching as you fill your lungs. Feel the way your abdominal muscles relax to allow full expansion of your lungs. Feel your diaphragm drop and loosen.

Now slowly exhale through your mouth until you feel like your lungs are empty, usually a count of eight. And repeat.

Feel how your diaphragm contracts to expel the air in your lungs. Feel your abdominal muscles tighten to maintain your upright posture. Feel the way your rib cage collapses gently around your deflating lungs, the slender bones cradling those infinitely important organs protectively. Feel your shoulders roll slightly on each exhale as tension eases in your neck, shoulders, upper arms and upper back.

Now, open your eyes. Did you feel it? Wasn't it amazing? It is extraordinary to know that your body does that every day of your life from the day you are born to the day you die without having to consciously think about it. But when you do think about it and take the time to *feel* it — it's absolutely mind-blowing!

Most people feel light-headed after a few minutes of this deep breathing; this is normal. Your body doesn't breathe as deeply when you are tense or active. Only when you are relaxed can you breathe as deeply as your body needs. You may feel a slight tingling in your extremities and this too is normal as more oxygen than your fingers and toes are used to is being sent to those capillaries.

Would you be surprised to find out you just centered yourself? Yes, it is true. You just *centered* yourself with that simple deep breathing method. In the same way that those who meditate begin their meditations.

This is the first step to learning Reiki for yourself. This sort of deep breathing and concentrating on how that air flows into your lungs and the mild relaxation and clarity of mind it offers. The next step is often the most fun, but can also be the most difficult for some people.

# Imagination Playtime (It's not just for kids)

Learning to use your imagination to help you focus your concentration is the next step toward learning Reiki. Yes, it's time to play with your imagination!

Interestingly enough, you actually use your imagination more often than you probably think. You know all those nagging little doubts you have about yourself, others or things you hear about? Even that skepticism you felt when you first started reading this book about Reiki? That's your imagination thinking up all the possible outcomes of a single, simple thought.

You probably know how to use your imagination, but allow me to walk you through the steps I think will make it easier for you to focus.

Find a place that is quiet and free of distractions and sit or lay down so that you are comfortable, but not likely to fall asleep. Now close your eyes and clear your mind as much as you can from outside distractions and thoughts for what you need to do later on in your day.

Concentrate and remember what a pot of boiling water looks like. You don't have to think about the stove it is on, just the pot and the water boiling inside. It's okay if you can't see the image clearly in your mind but the more clearly you can reconstruct the image, the more defined your focus will be.

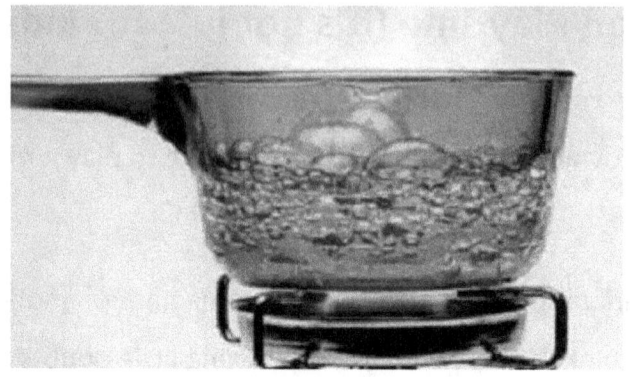

Do you see something in your mind? It may be flat or fuzzy, maybe a bit wobbly around the edges but that is perfectly fine. As long as you see something, you're doing great!

Once you have that image in your mind, the next step is to make it better, firm up the outline and bring it into better focus. You can do this by really thinking about it and bring the details back to your memory.

- What is the color of the part that holds the water?

- Make the pot in your mind the color you remember.

- Is the pot glass or metal?

- Does it have a texture on the outside surface of the pot? Are there any grooves, decorative enameling or is it completely smooth? Is it dull, shiny or something in between?

- What about the handle or handles of the pot. Does it have a single handle? Is it plastic, glass, metal or silicone?

- What shape is the handle? How thick is it? Are there any grooves in the handle to make it easy to hold? Is it riveted, welded or molded to the bowl of the pot?

Once you feel like you have remembered everything you can about that pot of water, open your eyes and look at the world around you. Just let your mind wander for a few minutes and let those synapses relax a little.

Let's expand on this exercise. Close your eyes. Bring everything you remember about your pot back to mind and sharpen that image in your memory. Can you see it? Does it look like you could reach out and touch it? You're doing very well! Now imagine more details to the picture in your mind.

- How much water is in the pot? Is it half-way up the side or just an inch below the rim?

- Is it boiling fast or slow?

- Can you imagine the sound of the water boiling?

- What does the boiling water smell like?

- Can you feel the heat radiating off the pot?

This is the step that will probably take you the longest in which to become proficient. Once you have that pot of boiling water pictured in your mind, you need to fix it in your mind so that you can call it up whenever you want. You can do that by describing it in vivid detail to someone else, recording it with a tape recorder, typing it out in a word-processing document or writing it down in a journal.

Most people can commit things to memory when they do three things with the information: see or read it, write it down, and hear it. This is why teachers will have power points up on a screen while they are giving a lecture and the student is taking notes. The student sees the words or pictures on the power point, they hear the instructor's words and they write those words down, allowing them to commit the lesson to memory. When you can listen to or read your description and picture it in your mind with no trouble, then you know the description is good.

Now that your description is vivid, you can go on to the next step of focusing. Bring your image to mind. You should be able to hear the water gurgling in the pot, the sound of the pot contracting or expanding as temperature changes occur and any sounds the heat source makes like the soft hiss of the gas flowing to fuel the flames on a gas stove or a slight ticking as electricity heats an element on an electric stove.

Imagine yourself leaning over the pot. You should be able to look into the pot and see the water boiling and the steam rising from the roiling surface. Breathe the steam in.

- How does it smell?

- Can you taste the metallic flavor of the chemical treatment of the water being released?

- You should be able to feel the difference in temperature as the steam rises to touch your face.

- Feel the gentle pressure of the steam as it causes your skin to react to its presence.

- Feel the moisture from the steam in your sinuses and maybe your lungs.

Excellent! It isn't completely necessary to imagine the pot of boiling water in this detail but the better you can see it, the easier it will be for you to use and utilize Reiki. This exercise will really help you to visualize the streams of energy flowing into and through your body.

You may still be skeptical about actually being able to see or feel this energy since most people consider energy as being without substance. Substance, as in something that can be felt and seen like the steam rising from your pot of boiling water, is energy that *can* be seen and felt.

What does this energy look like? It is different for each person who practices Reiki. There are many ways that the energy can look to you. You may see it as a distortion of color like oil on wet pavement, or a cloud of color like seeing something bright through a sheet of water. It might just be a spot of color brighter than anything around it.

What does this energy feel like? Again, there are so many ways that the body can interpret the sensations given off by this energy that it is nearly impossible to tell you how *you* will feel it. It may be a simple change in temperature, usually warmer but sometimes cooler. You might feel a change in pressure against your skin. It might tingle, though not painfully as when your foot or hand falls asleep. You might experience it as a vibration or even a sound. It might be a simple tone or a low or high harmonic tone. It may sound like a chant or song with both melody and harmony making it a collection of sounds. However you experience this energy, *believe* that you really did see, feel or hear what you saw, felt or heard.

Expanding your senses

Now that you've experienced this energy, let's go back to your pot of boiling water. Once you have that image in your mind, add some rice to the boiling water. Let it cook! See the rice grains moving in the water as they start to absorb the water. You can almost see how the bubbles form and roll to the surface to break and release a puff of steam. Lean in and smell the steam now. Do you remember how wonderful cooking rice smells?

Take a clean, clear glass and hold it in the steam. Watch as the steam condenses on the glass and makes it cloudy. Take the glass away and let the steam evaporate. The glass isn't clean anymore, is it? There is a film that dulls the clear glass. This is because some of the rice actually gets carried away with the steam and gives it that lovely smell.      Rice is food or nutrition for your body. If you don't get enough nourishment, you will find it difficult to function properly and can become malnourished.

Becoming malnourished can lead to illness that causes your body to malfunction and can even lead to death if it continues for too long. Getting the proper nutrition allows your body to function properly and makes it possible for you to live.

Consider that metaphor. Don't *think* about it, experience it. Let it fill your mind as you concentrate on every aspect of it: see it, smell it, hear it and feel it. Make it so real in your mind that you can reach out and touch it. Then learn from what you see.

This game of imagination will help you to focus your concentration just as feeling your breathing helped you center yourself. These are the beginning steps of learning to use Reiki and are a form of meditation in and of themselves. They will be used to allow you to enter into a relaxed state that encourages the flow of the life force energy through your body and takes care of those ripples and knots from the lines of energy that run throughout your body or someone else.

The next step to learning how to use Reiki and that life force energy is pretty fun and relaxing. Take a look and enjoy!

# Time to Veg Out!

You probably think I've gone crazy, huh? But I assure you, I haven't and this will help you start using Reiki for yourself.

This step is really called the Trance State. It has a lot of different names: Zoning, Spacing, Daydreaming, Fantasizing, Visualizing, and so forth. They all mean the same thing and you will eventually be able to slip in and out of this trance state whenever you want to.

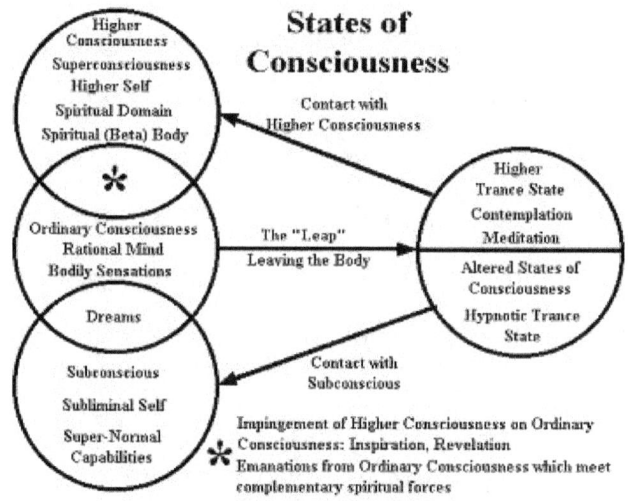

To reach this state, you'll use the deep breathing exercise we talked about earlier. You'll be using your imagination as well, but not to visualize a pot of boiling water.

Concentrate on your breathing. Breathe in for a count of four and out for a count of eight or more if you are able. With every exhale, feel your body relaxing. Don't force yourself to relax, just let it happen. Does it seem like it's taking forever to feel your body relax? That's okay, it will take as long as it takes for your muscles to relax completely; five, ten, fifteen minutes or more. Just continue concentrating on your breathing and those muscles will relax.

Once your body has relaxed, you can work on relaxing your mind. Don't try to get rid of all the thoughts running through your head. You won't be able to because the human brain is designed to continually process stimuli without conscious thought. Thoughts may come, but you can simply observe them and let them float away.

Think of it this way: you are standing in the middle of a crowded room, maybe a museum or shopping mall's food court – the noise you hear are your thoughts. Imagine all the conversations going on around you but you just can't understand them all at once. Your ears hear the words but there are so many coming in at once that your brain can only hear noise. Let your thoughts flow through your mind but don't try to interpret them at all. When you can let them flow without any of them catching your attention, imagine that the volume of those thoughts is diminishing until you can no longer detect them. Eventually, you will be able to imagine those thoughts no longer clamoring for attention. Once those thoughts no longer grab your attention, you will be able to silence your mind whenever you wish.

Smile more often

It can be difficult to relax fully if you are angry or upset about anything. Here is something I know will help. You know that when you are happy, you tend to smile, right? Did you also know that when you smile, the action itself tends to make you feel happy? It really does work. When you smile, you emit positive vibes that actually attract more positive things into your life.

Next time you're feeling sad or upset, smile. See how it makes you feel and watch good things come into your life. Did you know that when you use your imagination that you tend to look upward? Give it a try. Sit with your eyes straight ahead and close them. Now roll your eyeballs upward. If you look upward for thirty seconds to a minute, you will find that your imaginary pictures will sharpen and become stronger.

When your imagination turns on, *use* it. If you see something, concentrate on that image.

- What does it look like?

- What color is it? Is there a texture?

- How does light fall on the surface?

- Does it smell like anything? Is it a pleasant smell or a repulsive odor?

- Can you hear it? Is it musical or does it sound like some kind of animal or voice?

- Does it have a taste? Is it sweet, sour, bitter or salty?

Once you have spent a few minutes on this, open your eyes and focus on the world around you again. If you have time to do so, try it a few more times and you should feel yourself dropping into that trance more easily and deeper than you have before. If you practice this way for five to ten minutes a time several times a day for at least a week, you will master the technique. You will get to the point where you can flip your imagination on and off whenever you want, with time and practice. When this happens, you will find your imagination is highly active and quite vivid.

After you are comfortable with slipping in and out of that trance state, you might want to see if you can maintain that state of mind and still interact with the world around you. This will help you when you use Reiki both on yourself and on others if you choose to do that as well.

You might ask, "How can I be In The Zone and still move around and do things?" The answer is to practice doing just that. Put yourself into that trance state and decide that you will remain in that quiet mental and relaxed physical state. Don't worry about it too much if you find it difficult to retain that mental and physical relaxation when you first practice this skill. It is perfectly normal to have trouble with this the first several times you attempt it.

At first, you will want to remain sitting or lying down and just try to stay in that trance while you open your eyes and look at whatever is directly in front of you. What is the object you see? Does it look the same as if you weren't in that Zoned Out state? Recall how it feels when you touch it, but don't try to do that yet. Think about how it sounds or smells or tastes.

When you can retain that trance-like state and open your eyes to use your external senses easily, then you are ready to attempt moving while keeping a hold on that Spaced Out feeling. First, just move your eyes and then your head until you work your way up to moving your body while still feeling completely relaxed with your thoughts silent in your head.

As soon as you can move without dropping out of The Zone, try to walk through an open doorway. Take notice of how you feel and how the world seems to change as you walk from one room to the next. Feel how the ambient sensations change as you move through that doorway. Did you walk into a tense situation? Determine to have no expectation of the situation. Is it more calming than where you just came from? Does it make it more difficult or easy to retain that trance-like state? Try to describe the feelings you have so that someone else can understand it.

When you have moved through that door, feel free to go back to your normal state and examine those sensations. If you make this exercise a habit, you will eventually find it much easier to flip from one state to another in the depth required to sense the life force energy – and from there, manipulate it close up and from a distance.

# Seeing and Manipulating Reiki Energies

Up to this point we have talked about what Reiki is, how it can help you relax, reduce stress and increase your own energies as a wonderful side effect of using Reiki. Now we are going to discuss the actual use of Reiki.

Now that you know how to reach a super relaxed state, you will need to direct the flow of that life force energy that flows through you, me and every living, breathing thing in this world both animate and inanimate. After all, anything made from a natural substance such as stone, wood and metal will hold some amount of this life force energy.

Life force energy is such a mouthful, isn't it? Let's simplify it a little. This energy is also called Qi (pronounced *key*) or Chi (pronounced *chee*).  Now that you know how to see this Qi, you need to practice manipulating it.

Give it a try

By this time you should be practiced at sensing the Chi in any natural object, animal or person. You know that it can be moved, directed and otherwise manipulated. Now it's time to try your hand at it.

Let's begin with something simple like a blade of grass. You can drop into that trance-like state and feel the energy radiating from and flowing through that blade of grass. Once you feel that Qi, you can imagine putting your 'hand' *inside* that energy. Can you feel the energy inside that blade of grass flowing over, around, and through your hand? Move your hand back out and then repeat that exercise as many times as you have to so that you can recognize the energy that is responsible for the growth of the grass itself.

Feel the metabolism of each cell and try to find the unique energy field that is responsible for life itself. Examine the way that energy feels, sounds, smells, tastes and looks like. That signature line will be the same in everything, animal and person that you touch in this way.

This picture is of the energy running through a single leaf. Just imagine how it would feel to put your hand into such a dense flow of pure life force

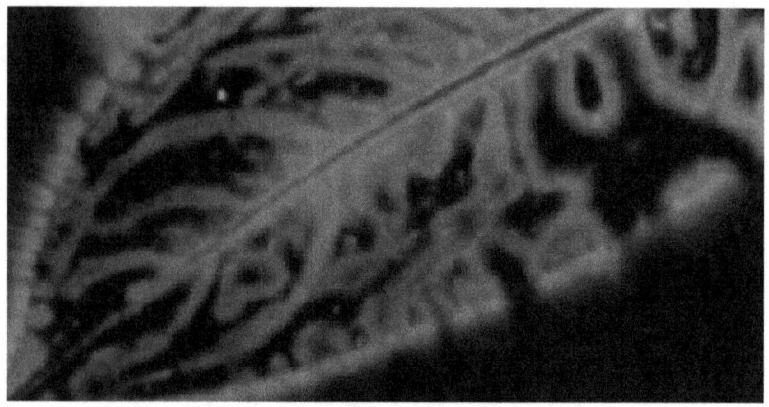

energy.

*That is Reiki!* That unique energy field, that 'signature' line of energy *is* Reiki. Now that you know what that unique line feels, looks, smells, tastes and sounds like, you can begin to manipulate it to do what your body needs it to do.

Manipulation of that life force energy is extraordinarily simple now that you have found that signature energy. You may feel more comfortable manipulating your Qi with both hands rather than just one. This is perfectly acceptable, simply place your hands atop one another or slightly overlapping in the most natural way for you.

Even if you don't necessarily "feel" anything, it is up to you to believe that such a life force energy exists.  You cannot always go by your five senses when it comes to supernatural things like this.  Know that Qi is real and determine to fully believe in the power of Reiki.

Breathe, relax your body and silence your mind as you put yourself into The Zone. Find that unique energy signature that controls your own life source. Place your palm on the crown of your head as if just resting your hand there. Let it rest there for as long as you feel necessary and visualize the energy flowing from your palm into the crown of your head. Imagine all the tension being soothed away as those ripples and knots in your energy flow are smoothed out so that the stream is swift and smooth once more.

Continue the process of placing your hand and visualizing the energy flowing into that spot before moving on to the next position until you have smoothed out all of the rough patches in your life force energy. Below is a list of the positions for your hand that cover the six chakras. For the two positions on your back, you will have to visualize the energy flowing from the back of your hand rather than your palm if you are unable to place your palms against your back.  Consult the diagram if you are unsure where to let your hands rest on your body.

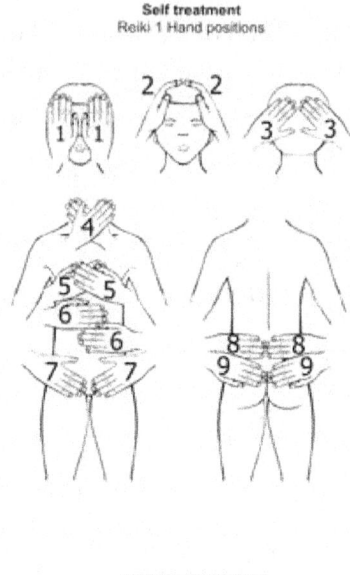

- The Crown Chakra. The crown of your head.

- The Third Eye Chakra. The forehead between the eyes often called the 'third eye'. This is where your pituitary gland is found. Or both eyes if using both hands with your thumbs overlapping above the bridge of your nose.

- The Throat Chakra. The occipital bulge at the back of your skull above the neck.

- The hollow at the base of your throat above the breastbone.

- The Heart Chakra. The center of your breastbone.

- The Solar Plexus Chakra. The diaphragm just below the breastbone.

- The navel, or bellybutton.

- The Sacral Chakra. The lower belly between your navel and pubic bone, this position is coincidentally associated to your bladder and sex organs.

- The small of your back at the base of the lumbar spine just over your kidneys.

- The Root Chakra. The sacral region of your spine, the plate of bones that lead to your tailbone. This site is a few inches below the previous site and just where the crevice between your buttocks begins.

Those are the areas you will feel the strongest flows and can manipulate the energy to smooth the flow easily. Manipulating the energy within the lower limbs is possible though there is no 'main' line of energy to position your hand over. If you have pain or discomfort in any joint or muscle in your buttocks, thighs, knees, shins, calves, ankles, feet or toes you can still ease those aches, pains or injuries through the manipulation of your Qi.

Simply lay your hand where you feel the need for relief and visualize the energy entering that area to soothe the aches, encourage blood flow to carry damaged tissue away and ease the knotting of the natural energy flowing through that area. Continue moving from one area to another until you feel that you have completed your task.

Look at the diagram on the next page to get an idea of how to cradle your ankle or foot to treat one or both. You can also do the same with your knees, thighs and calves; simply rest one hand on the front and the other on the back so that your energy can flow in both directions at once.

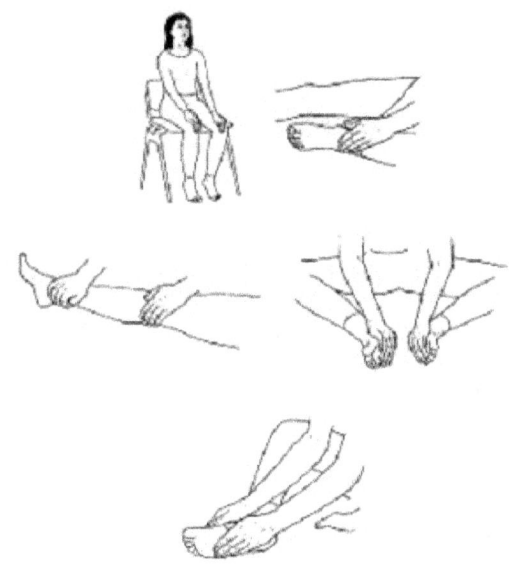

Once you are finished working from head to toe you should feel calm, relaxed, refreshed and revitalized with a better outlook on life, more energy and happiness overflowing your mind.

Doesn't it feel wonderful? It's amazing how great you feel even if you did begin as a skeptic. This method of 'energy healing' really does work if you remember that it requires *belief* that it will work. Believe it works and <u>then</u> you will receive it!

I leave you today hoping that I have offered you relief for the strains you find yourself under and with a better understanding of how you can affect your own mind and how your mind can affect your body and the energy that flows through it.

## Final Thoughts

Now that you know what Reiki is, how it works, how it can help you to relax, reduce stress and increase your energy, as well as how it feels to touch that universal energy flowing through you.

Your final lesson is simple. There are three symbols associated with Reiki that are usually given during the second stage of becoming a Reiki master, but they can be quite useful for you once you can touch and utilize your Reiki.

These symbols create a temporary connection between you and the person you are thinking about. Remember that Reiki is a benevolent energy and cannot cause harm.

The first symbol is the Distance Healing Symbol.

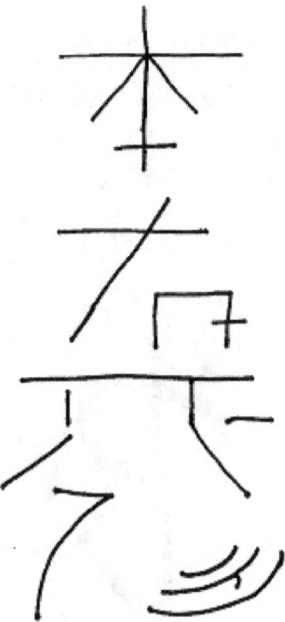

This symbol has been translated as meaning no past, no present, and no future. Quantum physics books like Lynne McTaggart's *The Intention Experiment,* shows us that there is no past, present or future. Everything is connected on the quantum level. Since everything is connected, there is no distance between you and me – no matter where we happen to be physically located. Everything is part of the same thing! Both past and future are illusions.

This symbol can be difficult to draw since it is so complex but it is mainly just straight lines. Eventually, with enough practice, you will be able to draw it with your fingers quickly and easily. Some people use a card and draw their fingers over the pattern while concentrating on the person they wish to connect with using Reiki.

You can use this energy that you have learned to see and touch. You can harmonize your intention for healing, peace and love with all that is. You can direct it toward a part of The All, which is that person.

The second symbol is the Clearing Symbol.

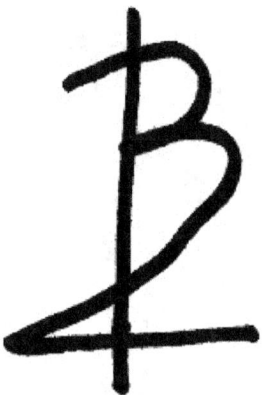

This is a very simple symbol and should not take you too long to learn to draw this with your fingers. This is one of the most often used symbols in Reiki and can be used nearly everywhere. As the cleansing symbol it represents healing. Before you can heal anything, you must brush away anything which is no longer useful. You can sometimes brush away negative energy as if it were dust or cobwebs tarnishing or clogging up the Reiki energy in yourself, someone you are performing Reiki on or even on a place you may find yourself.

The last symbol is the Power Symbol.

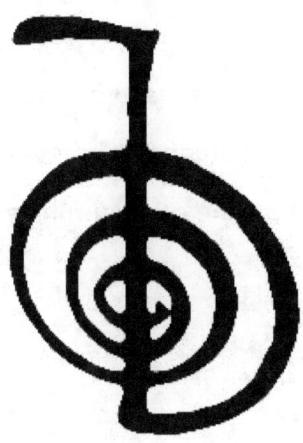

This symbol too is relatively simple to learn to draw with your fingers. The shape of a 7 that leads directly into an inward spiral. To use this symbol, simply see yourself empowering that which is already working, is already growing and is already good.

I hope that I have given you the information you were looking for. This is a time of change and transition in the healthcare system, and plenty of people are looking for alternative healing treatments over conventional treatments. The ancient healing method of Reiki is gaining momentum when it comes to such a healing avenue. It is simple, effective, and does not necessarily cost anything, as you can use Reiki on yourself.

If you utilize this universal life force energy within yourself to connect with other people, yourself, and the universe, you will find it much easier to relax, reduce your stress and increase your natural energy. Reiki works. Reiki will never cause harm. You and I and everyone and everything else in the universe is connected on the quantum level and are part of The All.

Sending Light and Love to ALL.

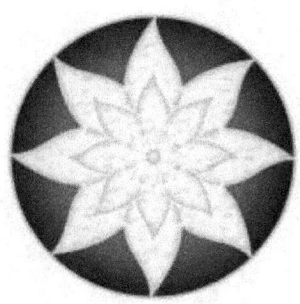

From Usui Mikao, founder of the Reiki technique, I offer you the Reiki Precepts:

*Just for today:*

*Do not be angry.*

*Do not worry.*

*Be grateful.*

*Work diligently.*

*Be kind to others.*

www.ingramcontent.com/pod-product-compliance
Lightning Source LLC
Chambersburg PA
CBHW070404290526
45790CB00004B/1629